I0435511

Chia Seeds For 30 Days: Discover How to Increase your Energy, Control Weight, Lower Cholesterol, and Reduce Inflammation

Copyright © 2016 by Tamira Wilson

This eBook contains information that is intended to help the readers be better informed consumers on their health. It is presented as personal thoughts and experience from the author. Always consult your doctor for your individual needs.

ACKNOWLEDGMENTS

To Raymond Wilson (husband), Tiara Murphy (Daughter), Cynthia Reid (Mother) for trying some of my weird, but healthy chia seed recipes I've made while taking a challenge to a healthier eating lifestyle. Also, to Tranny Reid (my brother), who always had a listening ear when I enthusiastically shared new recipes I made and who tried chia seeds for himself. Thanks family for your much love, support, and for jumping onboard and putting up with my craziness!

Table of Contents

INTRODUCTION

INTRODUCTION

Can anyone really survive off of chia seeds? I think you could…. mixed with just water. I'm sure you remember the old time chia pet that people were giving as gifts, which found notoriety in every household for the famous jingle "Cha Cha Cha Chia." Who would have ever thought these little seeds that grew sprouts from the chia pet was a superfood.

I personally experimented with chia seeds and added it to my diet as well as my husband's diet. I shared the benefits with my daughter as well, and she added some to her water. I would add a Tablespoon consistently to my husband's smoothies in the morning. He began losing weight (without going to the gym) and started receiving lots of compliments on how great he looked. People began asking him what he was doing, and he told some people the smoothies I had been making. Hahah……there was one person he told about the smoothie **he** made, and the person said, "I'm sure your wife had something to do with it." They both laughed and he agreed I was the one who started him on this chia seed diet and making the smoothies, which made him feel more energized on the job.

He didn't like how much weight he was losing, so he makes his own now and came up with his own concoction.

Let me just share a few of the following reasons why you should implement an intake of chia seeds in your diet:

Make you feel full faster: Great for dieting! Makes you feel full due their ability to absorb 10 times their water weight

Reduce food cravings: Helps with weight loss due to the fact of a reduction of craving bad foods or any food.

Keeps you hydrated: When chia seeds is mixed with water, it forms a gel, which helps keep the body hydrated. This is excellent for athletes or anyone who works out at the gym or those with heavy labor jobs.

No Need to Ground Up: Easily digested. Even easier than flax seeds!

Rich is Omega-3: This is great for those who suffer from heart disease or arthritis, as it is known that chia seeds have more Omega-3 than salmon, and helps protect against inflammation since it has a rich plant source of Omega-3.

Controls blood sugar: This is beneficial for diabetics because chia seeds have the ability to slow down how fast the body changes carbs into sugar.

Helps High Blood Pressure: Chia seeds are known to reduce blood pressure

Gluten Free: Beneficial for people who are suffering from gluten celiac disease because chia seed is a gluten free grain.

So there you have it! These are just a few benefits, but enough to consider including in your diet, which is why I'm challenging every reader to partake in a 30 day challenge to incorporate chia seeds into your diet any way you can. I have provided 30+ recipes in this book for ways you can include this in your diet. Whether you include it in your breakfast, lunch, dinner, snack or drink, you have the ability to improve your health.

Now…Are You Ready To Start Your Challenge? Well keep reading and thanks for purchasing my book. It may be helpful if you look through each recipe to plan ahead on how to prepare for one week. Enjoy and Cheers to a Healthier You!!

Why You Need To Do This? Getting just a few tablespoons of chia seeds a day provides enough recommended levels of phenolic anti-oxidants, minerals, vitamins and protein.

CHAPTER 1: CHIA BREAKFAST

TASTY CHIA OMLETTE WITH FETA CHEESE & SPINACH

QUICK MINI CHIA EGG MUFFINS

WHOLE WHEAT CHIA SEED PANCAKES

OATMEAL WITH A LITTLE CHIA

TASTY CHIA OMLETTE WITH FETA CHEESE & SPINACH

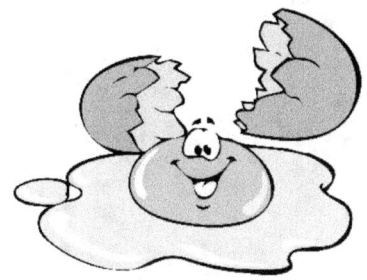

INGREDIENTS:

2 eggs

2 Tbsp. cup low fat milk

1 tsp Chia seeds

Cracked black pepper

1 tsp olive oil

1 oz fetta cheese, crumbled (or more to your liking)

½ cup baby spinach

INSTRUCTIONS

Beat the eggs together with milk, Chia seeds and black pepper. Set the mixture aside for about 10 minutes. Heat a small non-stick omelette pan with olive oil and pour the mixture into the pan. Tilt the pan around to ensure egg mixture completely covers the pan and cook under a medium heat until the omelette is almost cooked. Crumble the feta over the surface with the spinach and continue to cook until the spinach has slightly wilted. Fold the omelette in half and serve.

Tip: I used a little coconut oil & butter when cooking. Delicious!

QUICK MINI CHIA EGG MUFFINS

INGREDIENTS:

10 ounces fresh baby spinach, cooked

1 large Roma tomato, diced

4 whole large eggs

4 egg whites

1 medium Vidalia onion, diced

2 Tbsp. finely chopped fresh parsley

2 Tbsp. chia seeds

¼ tsp. sea salt

¼ tsp. freshly ground white pepper

INSTRUCTIONS

Preheat oven to 350 degrees F.

In a medium sized bowl, whisk eggs with egg whites. Add remaining ingredients; mix well to combine.

Prepare a muffin tin with nonstick baking spray. Pour egg mixture evenly into cups.

Bake for 30 minutes or until set. Remove from oven; set aside to cool.

Serve warm or place in the refrigerator for up to 5 days and serve for a quick breakfast or snack. My family loves these little babies to take on the go in the mornings off to work.

TIP: I add cheddar cheese to mine and make half plain without vegetables for my daughter.

WHOLE WHEAT CHIA SEED PANCAKES

INGREDIENTS :

2 Cups Whole Wheat Pancake Mix (Bob's Red Mill Pancake/Waffle)

Want gluten free pancake mix? Great! Try Bob's Red Mill! (Bob's Red Mill Gluten-Free Pancake Mix)

2 tsp sugar

2 eggs

1/4 cup water

3 Tbsp Chia Seeds

If you follow the directions on the bag, you don't have to use eggs. The eggs give the pancake more protein, a better crisp, and better taste!

INSTRUCTIONS

Mix together the eggs and pancake batter.

Stir in the water and Chia Seeds

Let the batter sit in the fridge for about 10 minutes.

While the batter is refrigerating, grease the skillet and heat on medium high.

Pour 1/3 cup of the batter into the prepared skillet.

OATMEAL WITH A LITTLE CHIA

INGREDIENTS:

1 Tbsp Chia Seeds

Milk/Almond Milk

Water

Butter (optional)

Brown Sugar (optional)

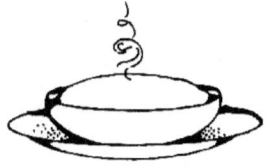

INSTRUCTIONS

Make oatmeal according to package. I use the good Old Fashioned Quaker Oats or Bob's Red Mill Steel Cut Oats when I want to eat healthier. When done, I add some chia seeds, a little butter and a dash of the brown sugar.

CHAPTER 2: CHIA LUNCH

EXCELLENT BRAIN POWER SALAD

CHIA CHICKEN BURGERS ON FOCCACIA BUNS

HEALTHY CHIA BEAN BURGERS

TASTY CAULIFLOWER AND CHICKPEA PATTIES WITH CHIA SEEDS

CHIA BRAIN POWER SALAD (Spinach, Salmon, Avocado and Blueberries)

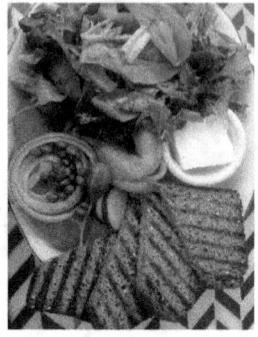

INGREDIENTS FOR SALAD

8 ounces smoked salmon, roughly chopped

1 avocado, peeled, pitted and diced

4 cups baby spinach (or mixed greens)

1/2 cup fresh blueberries

1/4 cup light feta or blue cheese crumbles

1/4 cup chopped walnuts (optional)

half a red onion, thinly sliced

honey chia seed vinaigrette (ingredients below)

HONEY CHIA SEED VINAIGRETTE INGREDIENTS:

1/3 cup olive oil

2 Tbsp. apple cider vinegar

1 Tbsp. chia seeds

1 Tbsp. honey

1/4 tsp. salt

INSTRUCTIONS

The Salad

Toss all ingredients together until combined. Drizzle or toss with vinaigrette.

The Vinaigrette

Whisk all ingredients together until combined and emulsified. Yummy!! This is one of my favorites. Keeps me energized focused. My husband says it's a weird flavor. Enjoy!

CHIA CHICKEN BURGERS ON FOCCACIA BUNS

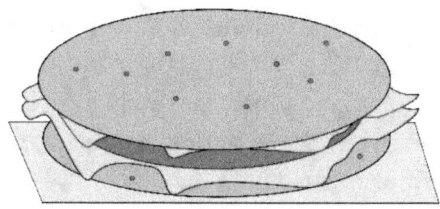

INGREDIENTS

½ kilo ground (minced) chicken

½ cup cooked brown rice or quinoa

½ cup grated carrot

½ cup grated zucchini

2 tbsp finely chopped parsley

2 – 3 tsp black Chia seeds

1 tsp sea salt, pepper (or to taste)

Olive or coconut oil (for cooking)

4 foccacia bread buns

Mayo, ketchup or tomato chutney

Tomatoes, greens and red onions

Cheese (optional)

INSTRUCTIONS

In a large bowl, mix the chicken, rice, carrot, zucchini, chopped parsley and Chia seeds well, and then form four patties. Heat a large frying pan on medium to medium-high heat, add oil and cook patties for about 5 minutes on each side. Reduce heat if browning too quickly. You can also cook on a grill. To serve, cut foccacia bread buns in half and spread a little mayo and ketchup (or tomato chutney) on bread. Place a piece of cheese, if using, on the bottom pieces then add a burger patty, tomatoes, greens and red onions if desired. Place top on and gently press down. Serve burger patties on a bed of mixed greens for a lighter meal. Tip: You can substitute chicken with ground (minced) beef, turkey, fish or prawns if desired.

HEALTHY CHIA BEAN BURGERS

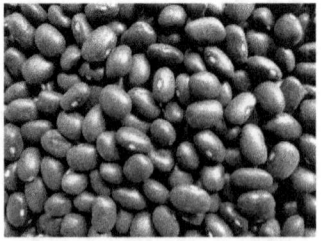

INGREDIENTS:

½ tsp dried Oregano

½ Cup Yellow Onion, minced

¼ Cup Navitas Naturals Chia Seed Sprouted Powder

1¼ Cup cooked Brown Rice

¼ Cup Nutritional Yeast

1 tsp Navitas Naturals Coconut Palm Sugar

2 Tbsp Wakame Flakes (Dried Sea Vegetable)

15 oz cooked black beans, unsalted

4 oz firm tofu, minced or crumbled fine

1 minced stalk Celery

1 minced Carrot

3 Tbsp organic Soy Sauce or Nama Shoyu

DIRECTIONS

Soak the wakame flakes in ½ cup warm water for about 20 minutes or until soft. Drain and set aside.

With a potato masher or the back of a fork, mash the black beans in a large bowl into a chunky puree. Mix in the remaining ingredients, one at a time. (Alternately, pulse ingredients together in a food processor). Form into 8-10 patties and refrigerate for about an hour.

Patties may be brushed with oil (can use coconut oil) and placed on a grill, or place into a well-greased frying pan and cooked over low heat for several minutes on each side. Makes 8-10.

TASTY CAULIFLOWER AND CHICKPEA PATTIES WITH CHIA SEEDS

INGREDIENTS:

1 medium cauliflower

250 gr of chickpeas, already cooked and drained

2 tsp of curry powder

Salt

Black pepper

10/12 tbsp of quick oats

2 tbsp of chia seeds

Extra virgin olive oil

INSTRUCTIONS

Cut cauliflower in florets and steam them. Once tender to your liking, place them in a food processor and reduce to cream. Blend chickpeas, leaving some chunks and mix them in a bowl with cauliflower cream, curry, salt, black pepper, chia seeds and oats. Add quick oats enough to have a soft mixture that you can handle to shape patties. Heat 2 Tbsp of olive oil in a non-sticking pan and cook patties, few minutes on each side until golden. Place them in dish with paper towel to absorb any oil (even if you used a small amount it's better to pat them dry). Serve patties still warm.

CHAPTER 3: CHIA SNACKS

VANILLA CHIA PUDDING

NUTELLA COCONUT CHIA PUDDING

LEMON & HONEY CHIA SEED MUFFINS

DELUXE CHOCOLATE MINI MUFFINS WITH CHIA SEEDS

CHIA COCONUT CARROT BREAD (GLUTEN-FREE)

UNIQUE BLACK BEAN CHOCOLATE CHILI CHERRY COOKIES

REFESHING CUCUMBER CHIA SEED SALAD

VANILLA CHIA PUDDING

INGREDIENTS:

3/4 cup almond milk, unsweetened (vanilla)

2 - 3 tsp maple syrup or honey

1 tsp pure vanilla extract

3 - 4 tbsp chia seeds

top with your favorite nuts, berries, fruit, coconut flakes (optional)

DIRECTIONS

Add all ingredients to a Mason jar or any container with a tight lid (I prefer glass), shake real good or stir and refrigerate for at least 6 hours or overnight. When ready to eat, stir and top with favorite toppings: nuts, berries, fruit, coconut flakes etc. Add extra milk to adjust to desired thickness. Add as little or as much honey/syrup to your liking.

Tip: I shake all ingredients in a mason jar and store in fridge and eat within 5 days. I've eaten this for my breakfast when in a rush or as a pre-workout meal.

NUTELLA COCONUT CHIA PUDDING

INGREDIENTS:

2 cups of Almond Milk

1/3 cup of Chia Seeds

1/4th cup of Shredded Coconut

2 tablespoons of Nutella

1/2 teaspoon of Vanilla

INSTRUCTIONS

Set out Nutella until it's room temp (or zap for 30 seconds in microwave). Combine Nutella, almond milk, chia seeds, coconut, and vanilla. Shake vigorously. Refrigerate 4+ hours. Top with fruit and fresh shredded coconut.

LEMON & HONEY CHIA SEED MUFFINS

INGREDIENTS:

1¾ cups all-purpose flour

¾ cup granulated sugar

2½ tsp. baking powder

¼ tsp. salt

¾ cup part-skim ricotta cheese

½ cup water

¼ cup olive oil

Zest of 2 lemons

2 tbsp. fresh lemon juice

1 egg

2 Tbsp. chia seeds

2 Tbsp. honey, melted

Cooking spray

INSTRUCTIONS

Preheat oven to 375 degrees Fahrenheit. Line a standard 12-cup muffin pan with cupcake liners and lightly spray them with cooking spray. Set aside.

In a large bowl, whisk together flour, sugar, baking powder, and salt.

In a medium bowl, mix together ricotta, water, olive oil, lemon zest, lemon juice, and egg.

Make a well in the center of the dry ingredients, pour the wet ingredients into the middle then mix together with a wooden spoon. Add the chia seeds then gently fold into batter.

Evenly divide batter into prepared muffin pan using a large scoop.

Bake for 16 minutes or until a toothpick inserted in the middle comes out clean.

Let cool for 5 minutes then with a pastry brush, gently brush melted honey onto the tops of the muffins.

Cool completely then enjoy!

Store in an airtight container for up to 7 days.

DELUXE CHOCOLATE CHIA MINI MUFFINS WITH CHIA SEEDS

INGREDIENTS:

1 cup all-purpose flour

1 cup white whole wheat flour

1 cup granulated sugar

3/4 cup semi-sweet chocolate chips

1/2 cup unsweetened cocoa powder

1 tsp. baking soda

1 Tbsp. black chia seeds

1 large egg

1 (6-oz) container low-fat vanilla yogurt

1/2 cup low-fat milk

1/2 cup canola oil

DIRECTIONS

Preheat oven to 400°. Spray a mini muffin pan with cooking spray (or use a 12-cup muffin tin and line with paper liner or spray with cooking spray).

Combine flours, sugar, chocolate chips, cocoa, baking soda and chia seeds in a large mixing bowl. In another small bowl, combine egg, yogurt, milk and oil with a whisk. Pour into the flour mixture. Stir to combine.

Scoop into muffin tins. Bake for about 15 minutes, or until springs back when touched on top.

CHIA COCONUT CARROT BREAD (GLUTEN-FREE)

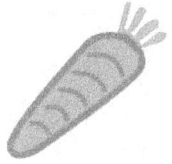

INGREDIENTS:

3 Tbsp. chia seeds

9 Tbsp. water

1 cup sugar

2 cups carrots, finely grated

1 ripe banana, mashed

1 cup olive oil

2 tsp. almond extract

3 cups Gluten-Free Cup 4 Cup Flour

1 tsp. baking soda

¼ tsp. baking powder

2 Tbsp. coconut flakes

1 tsp. sea salt

2½ tsp. ground cinnamon

INSTRUCTIONS

Preheat oven to 350 degrees F.

Combine chia seeds and water together in a medium bowl; mix well then let sit for 15 minutes.

Combine sugar, chia mixture, carrots and banana in a large bowl; mix well to combine. Set aside.

In a separate large bowl, combine remaining ingredients; mix well. Add sugar mixture to flour mixture; mix well to combine.

Transfer to 2 loaf pans.

Bake for 1 hour or until bread is set.

Remove from oven; set aside to cool before eating

UNIQUE BLACK BEAN CHOCOLATE CHILI CHERRY COOKIES

INGREDIENTS:

1 ½ cups black beans, very soft (or one 15 oz. can)

2 Tbsp. coconut oil (or ghee)

1/3 cup organic cocoa powder

1/4 tsp. coarse sea salt, plus more for sprinkling

1/4 tsp. cayenne pepper

1/3 cup maple syrup (or honey, agave)

2 Tbsp. chia seeds (or use 2 Tbsp. ground flax seeds OR 2 eggs)

1 tsp. vanilla extract

1/3 cup chopped dark chocolate (80% or higher)

1/4 cup chopped dried cherries (optional, or use dried cranberries)

DIRECTIONS

1. Preheat oven to 375°F. Line a baking sheet with good old parchment paper.

2. Mix chia seeds, maple syrup, and vanilla in a bowl and set aside. If using eggs, skip this step.

3. Place drained and well-rinsed beans, coconut oil, cocoa, salt and cayenne in a food processor and blend until well combined. Add maple syrup and chia mixture (or eggs) and pulse to incorporate. The batter will be quite liquid-y, but still hold together. Remove blade from the food processor and add chopped chocolate and cherries. Fold to incorporate.

4. Spoon cookie batter onto lined baking sheet. Using the back of the spoon, flatten top of cookies slightly, as they will

not spread when baking. Sprinkle with coarse sea salt (important!). Bake for 15 minutes until the edges are browning. Cool and eat. Store in the fridge.

REFESHING CUCUMBER CHIA SEED SALAD

INGREDIENTS (for two servings):

1 large cucumber, thinly sliced

1/2 yellow sweet onion, sliced

4 ½ tbsp. rice vinegar

1/2 tbsp. sweetener of choice (Stevia, Splenda, agave nectar or sugar)

Salt, to taste

½ tbsp. chia seeds

INSTRUCTIONS

Combine all ingredients except for chia seeds in a bowl and let sit for an hour. Right before serving, sprinkle with chia seeds on top. This is so refreshing! One of my favorites!

CHAPTER 4: CHIA SMOOTHIES

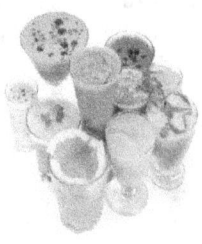

MANGO COCONUT AND YOGURT SMOOTHIE

EXCELLENT ANTIOXIDANT SMOOTHIE

NUTELLA COCONUT CHIA SMOOTHIE

TROPICAL CHIA SMOOTHIE

BANANA RASBERRY BLEND CHIA SMOOTHIE

SUPERFOOD CHIA GREEN SMOOTHIE RECIPE

ANTI-INFLAMMATORY SMOOTHIE WITH CHIA SEEDS

BANANA, STRAWBERRY & CHIA SEEDS SMOOTHIE

CRAZY WILD BLUEBERRY BANANA SPINACH POWER SMOOTHIE

MANGO COCONUT AND YOGURT SMOOTHIE

INGREDIENTS

1 cup diced mango flesh

½ cup lite coconut milk

½ cup plain yoghurt

½ cup skim milk or soy milk

1 tbsp white Chia seeds

1 tbsp honey

¼ tsp ground cinnamon

¼ tsp ground ginger

1 handful ice cubes

INSTRUCTIONS

Place all ingredients in a blender and blend until smooth. Serve in a tall glass with a straw.

EXCELLENT ANTIOXIDANT SMOOTHIE

INGREDIENTS:

1 cup frozen mixed berries

1/2 cup unsweetened pomegranate juice

1/2 cup water

1/2 tablespoon chia seeds

INSTRUCTIONS

Combine all ingredients in a blender, and mix until smooth.

Pour into your favorite glass & top of with an extra sprinkle of chia seeds if you want. This is one of my favorites!

NUTELLA COCONUT CHIA SMOOTHIE

INGREDIENTS

1/2 Chia Pudding from above

Handfull of Raspberries

1 Banana

Ice

DIRECTIONS

Using a blender, combine all of the above ingredients. Mix and enjoy!

TROPICAL CHIA SMOOTHIE

INGREDIENTS:

3/4 cup unsweetened coconut milk (the beverage next to the soy milk, not the canned kind)

1 cup frozen mango pieces

1 cup frozen pineapple pieces

1 banana

1 tablespoon chia seeds

INSTRUCTIONS

Pour coconut milk into a blender. Add mango, pineapple, and banana. Blend until smooth. Blend in chia seeds quickly. Enjoy right away, as chia seeds become gelatinous once they are wet.

BANANA RASBERRY BLEND CHIA SMOOTHIE

INGREDIENTS:

½ banana

½ cup raspberries

½ cup plain Greek yogurt

1 tablespoon chia seeds

1 scoop protein powder

½ cup water

½ teaspoon cinnamon

pinch of nutmeg

two handfuls ice - to taste

INSTRUCTIONS

Place all ingredients except for the ice in a high-speed blender and puree until smooth.

Add a handful or two of ice and pulse again until smooth.

Pour in a glass and enjoy!

SUPERFOOD CHIA GREEN SMOOTHIE RECIPE

INGREDIENTS:

2 cups cold water

2 handfuls spinach

1 kale leaf, medium

1/2 long English cucumber, sliced

1/2 any apple, chopped and not cored/seeded/peeled

2 Tbsp chia seeds

1/2 lemon (juice of lemon)

INSTRUCTIONS

In a blender, combine all ingredients and blend until smooth. If using a regular blender it is best to add the ingredients in the order listed above and press "pulse" on and off to get the blending process started. Then I usually hit "grate" and "liquefy" after. If you have a more powerful blender like I do (Nurti bullet), then the order doesn't matter. Drink immediately for best results!

ANTI-INFLAMMATORY SMOOTHIE WITH CHIA SEEDS

INGREDIENTS:

2 cups almond milk

2 Tbsp chia seeds

1 Tbsp raw honey

1/2 tsp cinnamon

1/2 tsp vanilla extract

DIRECTIONS

Blend all and enjoy! Cinnamon is a natural anti-inflammatory.

BANANA, STRAWBERRY & CHIA SEEDS SMOOTHIE

INGREDIENTS:

2 bananas, peeled & sliced

6 fairly large strawberries (almost 200g/7 ounces), hulled and diced

1 cup low fat milk or soy milk

2 Tbsps Greek yogurt (vanilla flavored is preferred)

2 tsps chia seeds as toppings

INSTRUCTIONS

(1) Hull and dice strawberries. Add to a blender. (2) Peel and slice bananas and add to the blender. (3) Then add milk and yoghurt with the bananas and strawberries. (4) Blend until smooth. Transfer to 2 glasses and top with chia seeds. Serve immediately.

CRAZY WILD BLUEBERRY BANANA SPINACH POWER SMOOTHIE

INGREDIENTS:

1/2 cup frozen blueberries

1/2 cup frozen strawberries, raspberries, or blackberries

1/2 frozen medium banana

1 cup Almond Breeze Unsweetened Vanilla Almond Milk

1 cup baby spinach

1 teaspoon chia seeds for topping, if desired

INSTRUCTIONS

Place all ingredients besides chia seeds into blender and blend until smooth. Add more almond milk if smoothie is too thick. Pour into a chilled glass, sprinkle with chia seeds and extra blueberries; enjoy!

CHAPTER 5: CHIA POWER WATER DRINKS

COOL GLASS OF LEMON CHIA SEED WATER

THIRST QUENCHER CHIA FRESCA

QUICK PRE-WORKOUT GREEN TEA AND CHIA SEED ENERGY DRINK

COOL GLASS OF LEMON CHIA SEED WATER

INGREDIENTS:

Several slices of lemons

1/2- 1 tbsp. chia seeds

INSTRUCTIONS

Mix all together

THIRST QUENCHER CHIA FRESCA

INGREDIENTS:

4 C. Cold Water

1 Medium Lemon, Half Juiced & Half Sliced

1/2 C. Fresh Fruit (I used Strawberries, Blackberries, and Pomegranate.)

1 Tbsp. Honey

2 Tsp. Chia Seeds

Directions:

Fill a large container with water. Add all of the ingredients and give it a good shake.

QUICK PRE-WORKOUT GREEN TEA AND CHIA SEED ENERGY DRINK

INGREDIENTS:

8 - 10 ounces filtered water

1 bag green tea (I used Numi Jasmine Green)

1 - 2 tablespoons chia seeds (depending on desired thickness)

INSTRUCTIONS

Bring water to a boil.

Let tea steep 3 - 5 minutes, then remove tea bag.

Add chia seeds and mix thoroughly.

Leave tea/chia seed mixture in the fridge for about an hour to cool.

Shake, drink, & work out!

TIP: I prepare this in advance so I can just grab in fridge before I work out during the week. I use within 5 days.

CHAPTER 6: CHIA FOR DINNER

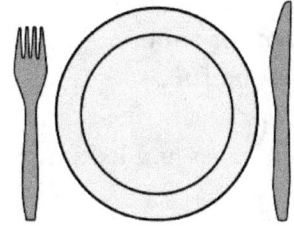

YUMMY CHIA CRUSTED SALMON

MEATBALLS WITH CHIA SEEDS

TASTY VEGAN CHIA CHILI

ROASTED CAULIFLOWER WITH CHIA SEEDS

YUMMY CHIA CRUSTED SALMON

INGREDIENTS:

½ cup finely chopped parsley

1 tsp lemon grated lemon zest (rind) (optional)

½ cup black and white Chia seeds

1 tsp sea salt and pepper (or to taste)

4 salmon fillets (skin removed)

2 Tbsp. olive oil (reserve 1)

INSTRUCTIONS

Place parsley, lemon zest, Chia seeds, salt and pepper in a blender and blend for 30– 60 seconds. Brush the fillets with reserved oil and divide the crust mixture evenly. Sprinkle over the top of each and press down gently to secure. Place the fillets in a baking dish, lined with baking paper and rubbed with 1 tsp oil. Bake in a 350F/180C oven for about 6 – 10 minutes. Then uncover and continue baking for 2 – 3 minutes or until cooked to your liking. Sprinkle with salt and pepper, if desired and serve with parsley leaves and lemon wedges

MEATBALLS WITH CHIA SEEDS

1 lb. ground beef (I like grass fed or no leaner than 85%)

2 Tbsp. organic tomato paste

2 cloves garlic, minced

2 t. your favorite Italian herbs

1 t. sea salt

1 t. ground pepper

2 T. chia seeds

2 t. 100% Pure Avocado Oil or coconut oil, for sauteing

DIRECTIONS

Combine all ingredients except the avocado oil in a large bowl and stir well with a fork.   Let rest for 5-10 minutes so the chia can expand.

Heat a large skillet over medium heat and add the avocado oil. Scoop 8 balls and pat into a round shape. Cook meatballs until brown, turning on at least 3 sides. Move meatballs to a plate to rest. (don't be alarmed if they are not cooked fully. They will be once finished cooking in the sauce. Drain all but 1-2 T. of oil from the pan.

EASY MARINARA

1 medium onion, diced

1 clove garlic, minced

sprig of fresh rosemary, chopped

2 T. white wine (or use juice of 1 lemon if no wine around)

1/2 c. beef or chicken stock (I use organic)

1 can organic diced tomatoes

1 can organic tomato sauce

1/2 tsp. sea salt

1/2 tsp. ground pepper

DIRECTIONS

Add diced onion to the large saute pan with the residual oil from cooking the meatballs. Saute until translucent, about 3-5 minutes. Add garlic and rosemary and cook 1-2 minutes. Add white wine and stock and scrape down any brown bits left at the bottom of the pan. Add the diced tomatoes, tomato sauce, salt, pepper, and stir well. Cook over medium heat until sauce begins to reduce and thicken, about 15-20 minutes. Reduce the heat to medium low and gently add meatballs to the outer edge of the pan. Cook 5-10 minutes, or until meatballs are cooked through to desired done-ness (10 minutes will ensure no pink inside).

TASTY VEGAN CHIA CHILI

INGREDIENTS:

1 Tsp oil

1-3 cloves garlic, minced (I used 1)

2 bell peppers, chopped

1 sweet onion, chopped

3 carrots, chopped

1 Tbsp cumin

3 Tbsp chili powder

pinch sea salt

pinch cayenne

1 can each: black beans, white kidney beans, red kidney beans (rinsed) (you can use 1 large mixed can)

1 can diced tomatoes with juice

2 tsp oregano

1 can organic mushrooms, drained

1 Tbsp unsweetened cocoa powder

2 Tbsp CHIA SEEDS

DIRECTIONS

In a large pot, add the EVOO and heat over medium. Add garlic, peppers, onion, carrot and sauté until everything is soft, approximately 5 minutes. Add the rest of the ingredients, cover, and cook for about 30-40 minutes on low to medium heat.

Optional: I add a dash of sugar and juice from 1 lime.

ROASTED CAULIFLOWER WITH CHIA SEEDS

INGREDIENTS:

1 tbsp. olive oil

a pinch of red pepper flakes

1 Tbsp. chia seeds

1 head cauliflower, broken into florets

salt + pepper, to taste

INSTRUCTIONS

Preheat oven to 400°F.

Heat olive oil and pepper flakes in a small saucepan over medium heat for about 3 minutes to infuse the flavor of the pepper into the oil. Set aside.

Line a rimmed baking sheet with foil. Transfer cauliflower to the baking sheet and drizzle with infused olive oil. Toss with tongs to coat. Sprinkle chia seeds over the cauliflower and add salt and pepper to taste.

Bake cauliflower for 20-30 minutes, or until softened and just beginning to brown.

BONUSES

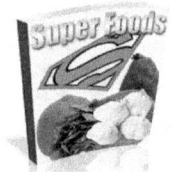

4 SUPERFOODS THAT HEAL

You may already know a few foods that are so packed with nutrients they're sometimes calls "superfoods." Acai and goji berries are good examples because they're rich in cancer-fighting antioxidants. But do you know about any of the following foods that may help prevent cancer, heart disease, and aid in digestive health?

Maca – High in protein and fiber, it contains more than 20 amino acids and helps increase your strength, energy, and endurance. Maca is a root vegetable and part of the cruciferous family, like kale and cabbage. You can purchase it in the U.S. mainly in its powder or extract form and add it to fruit smoothies, yogurt, or cereals. Look in any health food or drug store or on Amazon.

Spirulina – This is a type of freshwater blue-green algae that is 65% complete protein, greater than both red meat and soy. As little as 3 grams per day can help you increase energy and fight sickness. Buy it in capsules, powders, and flakes in health food stores but make sure it is "certified organic." It doesn't have the best taste, so add it to a smoothie or take as a supplement per directions on the bottle.

Kohlrabi – You get plenty of potassium, vitamin C, and fiber out of this antiviral vegetable, which is a blend of cabbage, turnips, and radishes. Find them at your farmer's market or grow them at home. To eat them, try pickling the bulbs or sauteing them.

Chia – Yes, the same Chia Pet commercial seeds are healthy and edible. You can get as much fiber out of chia as you can from your bowl of oatmeal. It also has plenty of iron, calcium, and omega 3s. Buy it in stores such as, Walmart, the Vitamin Shoppe, and GNC. It blends well in soups, salads, stir-fries, and cereal.

Hi, I'm Tamira Wilson, and I'm a Lifestyle & Wellness Coach and love helping individuals keep balance of Mind, Body, and Spirit while helping them achieve success in their health, finances, business, and relationships.

THANK YOU FOR DOWNLOADING AND INVESTING IN MY BOOK

As my way of saying thanks, I have an awesome FREE eBook, "Get Fit, Get Healthy", waiting for you. All you need to do is register at me site:

http://www.fitandsexyafter40.com

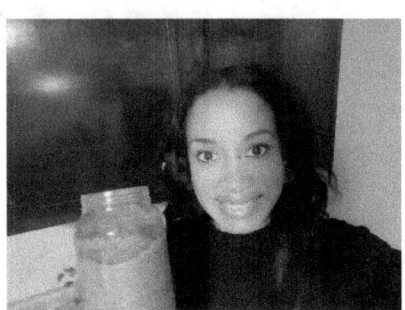

I hope you enjoyed reading this book and hope you'll enjoy the recipes. Can I ask a HUGE favor? It would mean so much to me if you could leave a helpful review with a few kind words on Amazon. Just go to www.amazon.com, and type in title of my book "Chia Seeds for 30 Days" and look for the link to leave a review. I'd love to hear your thoughts about the book. Thanks so much! I really appreciate it!

Remember….You got what it takes to be and achieve whatever it is you want in life.

Now, Go and Be Great at Something!

--Tamira Wilson

Staying Fit and Sexy After 40

support@fitandsexyafter40.com